Preserving memory

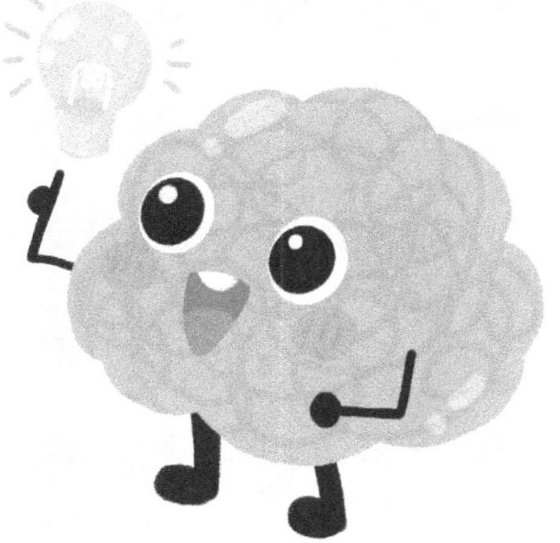

Preserving memory: how to prevent Dementia.

Sarah . P. Strum

Copyright

Dedication

This book is dedicated to you dear reader .

Content

Introduction

Evelyn lived in a curious little town settled in the midst of moving slopes and lavish plant life. Evelyn's vibrant spirit, infectious laughter, and unwavering kindness to others made her a household name. She went through her days keeping an eye on her nursery, chipping in at the neighborhood public venue, and imparting stories to companions over cups of steaming tea. Be that as it may, one game changing day, Evelyn's reality was profoundly affected when she got some disrupting news from her primary care physician. The doctor gently informed Evelyn, following a series of cognitive tests, that she had a genetic predisposition to develop dementia later in life. The news sent shockwaves through

Evelyn's heart, filling her with dread, vulnerability, and a profound feeling of trouble. Decided not to allow dread to direct her future, Evelyn sincerely committed to herself that she would do everything possible to keep dementia from grabbing hold of her psyche and denying her of the lively life she treasured so truly. With relentless assurance and a dauntless soul, Evelyn left on an excursion of disclosure, searching out each conceivable road for safeguarding her mental wellbeing and prosperity. Outfitted with information and directed by her PCP's proposals, Evelyn embraced an all encompassing way to deal with dementia counteraction. She embraced a cerebrum sound eating regimen wealthy in organic products, vegetables, entire grains, and omega-3 unsaturated fats, supporting her mind with the supplements it expected to flourish. She set out on an ordinary work-out everyday practice, integrating energetic strolls, yoga meetings, and dance classes into her day to day plan, stimulating her body and brain with each euphoric development. In addition, Evelyn placed a high value on getting enough quality sleep, designing a tranquil bedtime routine that included calming music, herbal tea, and methods of relaxation to encourage sound sleep. She participated in animating exercises, for example, perusing, crossword riddles, and learning new dialects, keeping her psyche sharp and lithe with each new test. In particular, Evelyn cultivated profound associations with her friends and family, encircling herself with chuckling, love, and friendship constantly. Years passed, and as Evelyn effortlessly explored the exciting bends in the road of life, she found comfort in the information that she was doing all that could be within reach to protect her mental wellbeing and save her valued recollections. As time passes, she felt a recharged feeling of imperativeness, lucidity, and reason flowing through her veins, directing her towards a future loaded up with vast potential outcomes and endless euphoria. So, in spite of everything, Evelyn triumphed over the gloom of dementia and became a shining example of hope and inspiration to everyone she met. Her story filled in as a demonstration of the force of strength, assurance, and enduring confidence despite misfortune, demonstrating that with the right outlook and backing, the sky is the limit. As the sun set into the great beyond, giving occasion to feel qualms about its brilliant beams the world beneath, Evelyn stood tall and glad, her heart overflowing with appreciation for the valuable endowment of life and the vast expected that lay ahead. Furthermore, at that time, she knew with steadfast sureness that her process was not even close to finished - for the best experience of all looked for her not too far off, enticing her forward with great enthusiasm and a commitment of vast conceivable outcomes yet to be found.

What is Dementia?

Dementia is a neurological condition described by a decrease in mental capability that slows down day to day exercises. It influences different mental capacities like memory, thinking, thinking, judgment, language, and conduct. While dementia is frequently connected with maturing, it's anything but a typical piece of the maturing system. Alzheimer's sickness is the most widely recognized kind of dementia, however there are different sorts also, including vascular dementia, Lewy body dementia, and frontotemporal dementia.

The effect of dementia on people and society is significant. Dementia can make it hard for people to be independent, do the things they need to do every day, and talk to other people. It can create sensations of turmoil, dissatisfaction, and seclusion, influencing one's personal satisfaction and profound prosperity. As the condition advances, people might require expanding levels of care and backing, overburdening family parental figures and medical services frameworks.

According to a cultural point of view, dementia presents critical financial and medical services troubles. The expenses related with really focusing on people with dementia are significant, including clinical costs, long haul care administrations, and lost efficiency due to providing care liabilities. Also, dementia puts tension on medical care frameworks, prompting expanded interest for particular administrations and assets. As the worldwide populace keeps on maturing, the predominance of dementia is supposed to rise, further featuring the significance of tending to this general wellbeing challenge.

Counteraction assumes an essential part in tending to the developing weight of dementia and advancing in general cerebrum wellbeing. By embracing way of life changes and executing preventive measures, people might possibly decrease their gamble of creating dementia and keep up with mental capability as they age. Here are a few key justifications for why counteraction is significant and the expected advantages of way of life changes:

1. **Lessening Chance Factors:** Many gamble factors for dementia, like hypertension, diabetes, heftiness, and smoking, are modifiable through way of life changes. By tending to these gamble factors from the beginning, people can bring down their endanger of creating dementia further down the road.

2. **Postponing Onset:** Way of life changes can assist with deferring the beginning of dementia, permitting people to appreciate

better mental capability and freedom for a more extended period. Over time, even modest changes in lifestyle habits like regular exercise and eating well can have a big effect on brain health.

3. **Further developing Generally Health**:

Changes in one's lifestyle that are good for the brain also help with one's overall health and well-being. For instance, normal activity can work on cardiovascular wellbeing, diminish the gamble of persistent illnesses, and improve mind-set and rest quality.

4. **Improving Nature of Life**: A healthy lifestyle for the brain can improve memory, concentration, problem-solving abilities, emotional resiliency, and other aspects of daily life. This can convert into more prominent freedom, efficiency, and fulfillment throughout everyday life.

5. **Giving Individuals Power**: Individuals can actively manage their own health and well-being by providing them with information and tools to prevent dementia. This feeling of strengthening can inspire people to roll out good improvements and keep up with sound propensities over the long haul.

6. **Decreasing Parental figure Burden**: Forestalling or postponing the beginning of dementia can likewise help parental figures and families by decreasing the weight of providing care liabilities. Caregivers may experience reduced stress and improved quality of life by promoting brain health and independence in older adults.

Generally speaking, the significance of counteraction couldn't possibly be more significant in tending to the worldwide test of dementia. By advancing mindfulness, instruction, and admittance to assets, we can engage people to make proactive strides towards protecting mental capability and advancing cerebrum wellbeing over the course of life.

Chapter 1

Understanding Dementia

- ## What is Dementia?

Dementia is an expansive term used to depict a decrease in mental capability that slows down everyday exercises. It's anything but a particular infection yet rather a gathering of side effects related with different hidden conditions.

The most prevalent forms of dementia are:

1.**Alzheimer's Illness**: Alzheimer's sickness is the most widely recognized reason for dementia, representing roughly 60-80% of cases. It is described by the aggregation of strange protein stores in the mind, prompting the ever-evolving weakening of synapses and mental capability. Side effects ordinarily incorporate cognitive decline, disarray, trouble with language and correspondence, and changes in conduct and character.

2.**Dementia Vasculare**: Vascular dementia happens when impeded blood stream to the mind harms synapses, frequently because of stroke or little vessel sickness. The side effects of vascular dementia can change contingent upon the area and seriousness of the harm however may incorporate issues with memory, consideration, arranging, and association.

3. **Lewy Body Dementia**: Lewy body dementia is portrayed by the presence of

unusual protein stores called Lewy bodies in the cerebrum. It imparts side effects to both Alzheimer's illness and Parkinson's sickness, including mental impedance, development troubles, mind flights, and variances in sharpness and consideration.

4. **Frontotemporal Dementia (FTD):** Frontotemporal dementia alludes to a gathering of issues portrayed by moderate harm to the front facing and transient curves of the cerebrum. Rather than affecting memory, it primarily affects personality, behavior, and language. Side effects might remember changes for social way of behaving, impulsivity, language challenges, and leader brokenness.

5. **Blended Dementia:** Blended dementia alludes to the presence of numerous sorts of dementia pathology in the cerebrum, like a mix of Alzheimer's sickness and vascular dementia. Mixed dementia is a common condition, especially in older people.

6. Different Sorts: There are a few other more uncommon sorts of dementia, including Parkinson's illness dementia, Huntington's infection, Creutzfeldt-Jakob sickness, and others. Each kind of dementia has its own unmistakable highlights, movement, and fundamental causes.

It's vital to take note of that while each sort of dementia has special qualities, there can likewise be cross-over in side effects, and determination can be mind boggling. Moreover, a few people might encounter a combination of side effects from various kinds of dementia. Early finding and proper administration are essential for advancing personal satisfaction and giving fitting consideration and backing to people living with dementia.

- Side effects of dementia

The side effects of dementia can differ contingent upon the basic reason and the phase of the condition. Notwithstanding, there are a few normal side effects that are frequently connected with dementia. These may include:

1. **Cognitive decline**: One of the most common signs of dementia is forgetfulness, especially of recent information or events. People may more than once pose similar inquiries or fail to remember arrangements, names, and significant dates.

2. **Trouble with Language and Correspondence**: Individuals with dementia might experience difficulty tracking down the right words, following discussions, or figuring out complex guidelines. They may likewise battle with composing or experience issues communicating their thoughts intelligently.

3. **Poor judgment and ability to make decisions**: Dementia can influence an individual's capacity to settle on good decisions and choices. This might appear as poor monetary administration, dangerous ways of behaving, or trouble in surveying circumstances and outcomes.

4. **Bewilderment and Disarray**: People with dementia might become bewildered and confounded finally, spot, and individual. They might experience difficulty perceiving natural environmental factors or tracking down their direction home, even in recognizable conditions.

5. **Changes in Mind-set and Conduct**: Dementia can prompt emotional episodes, unsettling, peevishness, and unresponsiveness. People might encounter quick changes in feelings or display socially unseemly ways of behaving. They may likewise pull out from social exercises and

lose interest in side interests or exercises they once delighted in.

6. **Trouble with Undertakings and Exercises**: Performing regular assignments and exercises might become trying for people with dementia. This can incorporate challenges with prepping, cooking, driving, or overseeing drugs.

7. **Disabilities in Motor Skills**: A few kinds of dementia, for example, Lewy body dementia and Parkinson's illness dementia, can cause development troubles, quakes, firmness, and issues with equilibrium and coordination.

8. **Changes in character**: Dementia can modify an individual's character, prompting changes in demeanor, interests, and social connections. People might turn out to be more uninvolved, removed, or disinhibited in their way of behaving.

It is essential to keep in mind that the signs and symptoms of dementia can differ from person to person and may get worse over time as the disease progresses. Early finding and fitting administration are critical for tending to side effects, expanding personal satisfaction, and offering help for people living with dementia and their guardians. On the off chance that you or somebody you know is encountering side effects of dementia, counseling a medical services proficient for assessment and guidance is significant.

Age, location, and demographics of the population all have an impact on the prevalence of dementia. Notwithstanding, dementia is a worldwide wellbeing worry that influences a large number of individuals around the world. Here are a few central issues with respect to the commonness of dementia:

1. **Worldwide Impact**: As per the World Wellbeing Association (WHO), an expected 50 million individuals overall were living with dementia in 2020. This number is projected to increment to 152 million by 2050 because of populace maturing and other segment patterns.

2. **Territorial Variations**: The commonness of dementia fluctuates altogether among districts and nations. Because of longer life expectancies and improved healthcare infrastructure for diagnosis and reporting, countries with high incomes typically have higher rates of dementia. Be that as it may, the predominance is additionally expanding in low-and center pay nations as populaces age and ways of life change.

3. **Age-related Risk**: Dementia is more normal in more seasoned grown-ups, with the gamble expanding essentially with age. While dementia can happen in more

youthful grown-ups, it is considerably less normal. After the age of 65, the prevalence of dementia roughly doubles every five years.

4. Influence on Maturing Population: As the worldwide populace keeps on maturing, the weight of dementia is supposed to significantly develop. Maturing populaces in numerous nations, joined with longer futures, are adding to the rising pervasiveness of dementia around the world.

5. Influence on Medical care Systems: Dementia presents critical difficulties for medical services frameworks, parental figures, and society in general. The condition requires long haul care and backing, overburdening medical services assets and family parental figures. Tending to the developing pervasiveness of dementia requires thorough techniques for counteraction, early discovery, and the board.

6.General Wellbeing Priority: Numerous nations and international organizations have given dementia top priority as a public health concern because of its rising prevalence. Endeavors are in progress to bring issues to light, further develop admittance to finding and treatment, and backing examination into preventive measures and viable mediations.

The prevalence of dementia as a whole is a serious issue that has far-reaching repercussions for individuals, families, and society as a whole. Tending to this challenge requires an organized and multi-layered approach that incorporates counteraction, early recognition, support for guardians, and progressing exploration to more readily grasp the basic causes and systems of the condition.

- **Basic causes and hazard factors related with dementia.**

Damage to brain cells impairs their ability to communicate with one another, resulting in dementia. This harm can result from different basic causes and chance variables. Here is an outline:

1. **Alzheimer's Disease**: The most well-known reason for dementia is Alzheimer's sickness, which includes the aggregation of strange protein stores in the mind, including beta-amyloid plaques and tau tangles. These stores impede ordinary cell capability, prompting the demise of synapses and the dynamic loss of mental capability.

2. **Factors Associated with the Vasculature**: Vascular dementia is brought about by diminished blood stream to the cerebrum, frequently because of conditions like stroke, little vessel illness, or hypertension. Brain cell death and cognitive decline can result from damage to blood vessels in the brain.

3. **Lewy Bodies and Parkinson's Disease**: Lewy body dementia is portrayed by the presence of strange protein stores called Lewy bodies in the cerebrum. These deposits interfere with normal brain function and are linked to dementia symptoms and Parkinson's disease-like movement problems.

4. **Frontotemporal Disorders**: A group of conditions known as frontotemporal dementia (FTD) are characterized by damage to the frontal and temporal lobes of the brain. This harm can result from different hidden causes, including

hereditary transformations, protein anomalies, or different elements.

5. **Hereditary Factors:** A few types of dementia, for example, beginning stage Alzheimer's sickness and particular sorts of FTD, have a hereditary part. People with a family background of dementia might be at expanded hazard of fostering the actual condition, albeit hereditary factors alone are seldom the sole reason for dementia.

6. **Way of life Factors:** Dementia risk can be exacerbated by certain health conditions and lifestyle choices. These incorporate smoking, over the top liquor utilization, stoutness, diabetes, hypertension, elevated cholesterol, and a stationary way of life. Embracing a sound way of life and dealing with these gamble elements can assist with diminishing the gamble of dementia.

7. **Natural Factors:** Openness to natural poisons, like weighty metals or certain

synthetics, may build the gamble of dementia. Furthermore, horrible cerebrum wounds, for example, those supported in mishaps or sports-related wounds, can build the endanger of creating dementia sometime down the road.

8. Age: Old age is the single most serious gamble factor for dementia. While dementia can happen in more youthful grown-ups, it is considerably more considered normal in more established age, with the gamble expanding essentially after the age of 65.

In general, dementia is a complicated condition with numerous risk factors and underlying causes. While some gamble factors, like age and hereditary qualities, can't be transformed, others, for example, way of life decisions and ailments, are modifiable. Individuals may be able to reduce their risk of developing dementia and maintain cognitive function as they age by addressing modifiable risk factors and adopting a lifestyle that is beneficial to the brain.

Chapter 2

Lifestyle Factors and Brain Health

- **The significance of lifestyle choices in preserving brain health.**

Way of life factors assume a urgent part in keeping up with mind wellbeing and decreasing the gamble of mental degradation and dementia. Taking on sound way of life propensities can advance brain adaptability, the mind's capacity to shape new associations and adjust to changes, and safeguard against age-related mental deterioration.

This is the way different way of life factors add to cerebrum wellbeing:

1. Actual Activity: Ordinary actual work has been displayed to have various advantages for mind wellbeing. Practice increments blood stream to the cerebrum, advances the arrival of synapses that help temperament and perception, and animates the creation of development factors that advance the development and endurance of synapses. Particularly, aerobic exercise has been linked to improvements in memory, attention, and cognitive function.

2. Sound Diet: For brain health, a well-balanced and nutritious diet is essential. Consuming an eating regimen wealthy in natural products, vegetables, entire grains, lean proteins, and solid fats gives fundamental supplements, cell reinforcements, and phytochemicals that help cerebrum capability and safeguard against oxidative pressure and irritation. Diets, for example, the Mediterranean eating regimen, which stress entire food varieties and sound fats, have been connected to a decreased gamble of mental degradation and dementia.

3. Mental Stimulation: Taking part in intellectually animating exercises, like perusing, puzzles, games, mastering new abilities, and mingling, can assist with keeping up with mental capability and advance brain adaptability. These exercises challenge the cerebrum, reinforce brain associations, and assemble mental save, which can help make up for age-related changes and safeguard against mental degradation.

4. Social Engagement: Keeping up with social associations and taking part in friendly exercises is significant for mind wellbeing. Social association invigorates the cerebrum, decreases pressure and wretchedness, and advances close to home prosperity. Support and opportunities for intellectual engagement are provided by strong social networks, which can assist in maintaining cognitive function and guard against loneliness and isolation, which are risk factors for cognitive decline.

5. Quality Sleep: Sufficient rest is fundamental for cerebrum wellbeing and mental capability. During rest, the cerebrum combines recollections, clears poisons and side-effects, and reestablishes energy levels. Ongoing lack of sleep has been connected to mental disability, mind-set unsettling influences, and an expanded gamble of dementia. Focusing on great rest cleanliness, for example, keeping a normal rest plan, making a loosening up sleep time schedule, and establishing an agreeable rest climate, can uphold mind wellbeing.

6.   **Stress Management**: Constant pressure can inconveniently affect mind wellbeing and mental capability. Delayed openness to push chemicals, like cortisol, can harm synapses, impede memory and learning, and increment the gamble of mental deterioration and dementia. The effects of stress on the brain can be lessened and overall well-being can be improved by practicing stress-reduction techniques like mindfulness, meditation, deep breathing, and relaxation.

Maintaining cognitive function, promoting neuroplasticity, and lowering the risk of cognitive decline and dementia are all benefits of living a brain-healthy lifestyle that includes regular physical activity, a nutritious diet, mental stimulation, social engagement, quality sleep, and stress management. By pursuing positive way of life decisions, people can uphold mind wellbeing and streamline mental capability over the course of life.

- **The effect of diet, exercise, rest, and stress the board on mental capability.**

1. Diet:

- **Supplement Intake:** Brain health and cognitive function are supported by a well-balanced diet high in nutrients like omega-3 fatty acids, antioxidants, vitamins (especially B vitamins), and minerals like zinc and magnesium. These supplements assume parts in synapse union, energy digestion, and neuroprotection.

- **It has anti-inflammatory properties**: Certain food sources, like natural products, vegetables, entire grains, and solid fats, have mitigating properties that might diminish aggravation in the cerebrum, which is related with mental degradation and dementia.

- **The Brain-Gut Axis**: Through the gut-brain axis, the gut microbiota can influence brain function. A solid eating regimen that supports stomach wellbeing, like one high in fiber and matured food sources, may emphatically influence mental capability and state of mind.

2. Exercise:

- **Cerebrum Blood Flow**: Actual work further develops blood stream to the mind, conveying oxygen and supplements fundamental for ideal mental capability. Growth factors that encourage the development of new brain cells and neural connections are also sparked by exercise.

- **Neuroplasticity**: Ordinary activity upholds brain adaptability, the cerebrum's capacity to adjust and revamp in light of encounters and upgrades. This can improve learning, memory, and mental adaptability.

- **Temperament Regulation**: Practice advances the arrival of synapses, for example, serotonin and endorphins, which further develop mind-set and decrease pressure and nervousness. Positive mind-set states are related with better mental execution.

3. Sleep:

- **Consolidation of Memory**: Rest assumes a basic part in memory solidification, the cycle by which recently gained data is moved from present moment to long haul memory. Sufficient rest, especially during the sluggish wave rest stage, upgrades memory maintenance and learning.

- **Mind Cleansing:** During rest, the glymphatic framework in the cerebrum cleans up poisons and byproducts, including beta-amyloid plaques related with Alzheimer's sickness. Disturbed rest designs or lacking rest might weaken this freedom instrument and increment the gamble of mental deterioration.

- **Close to home Regulation:** Quality rest upholds close to home guideline and strength, lessening the effect of pressure and gloomy feelings on mental capability. Lack of sleep, then again, can prompt touchiness, temperament swings, and weakened independent direction.

4. Stress Management:

- **Hormonal Balance**: Ongoing pressure enacts the body's pressure reaction framework, prompting the arrival of stress chemicals like cortisol. Delayed rise of cortisol levels can weaken mental capability, especially memory and leader capability.

- **Neuroprotection:** The negative effects of stress on the brain can be reduced through stress management strategies like mindfulness, meditation, and exercises in deep breathing. These practices advance unwinding, decline cortisol levels, and backing brain adaptability and mental strength.

- **Further developed Adapting Skills**: Successful pressure the executives procedures further develop adapting abilities and critical abilities to think, empowering people to all the more likely explore testing circumstances and keep up with mental capability under pressure.

In outline, diet, exercise, rest, and stress the executives significantly affect mental capability. By embracing solid way of life propensities and focusing on these key variables, people can uphold mind wellbeing, upgrade mental execution, and lessen the gamble of mental degradation and dementia.

- **The significance of mental excitement and social commitment.**

Social interaction and mental stimulation are crucial for preserving cognitive function and brain health as a whole. Here's the reason they are significant:

1. Stimulation of the mind:
- **Neuroplasticity**: Mental feeling difficulties the mind and advances brain adaptability, the cerebrum's capacity to frame new associations and adjust to changes. Learning new skills, puzzles, games, and intellectually stimulating activities like reading strengthen neural pathways and improve cognitive function.

- **Mental Reserve**: Mental feeling fabricates mental save, a defensive variable that empowers the cerebrum to endure age-related changes and pathology. People with more elevated levels of mental save might encounter milder mental side effects and a decreased gamble of dementia, even within the sight of cerebrum pathology.

- **Memory and Learning**: Memory, attention, and learning abilities all benefit from regular mental stimulation. Exercises that require dynamic commitment and critical thinking, for example, crossword riddles or learning an instrument, practice mental cycles and backing memory maintenance and review.

2. Social interaction:

- **Mind Health**: Social commitment has been connected to better mental capability and a diminished gamble of mental deterioration and dementia. Cooperating with others invigorates the cerebrum, advances the arrival of synapses that help temperament and comprehension, and diminishes pressure and sorrow.

- **Close to home Support**: Social associations offer close to home help and buffering against the adverse consequences of stress. Solid informal organizations offer open doors for sharing encounters, getting support, and encouraging a feeling of having a place and reason.

- **Mental Stimulation**: Social connections include complex mental cycles like point of view taking, compassion, and social discernment. The brain is challenged by group activities, collaborative projects, and conversations. These activities also encourage cognitive flexibility, empathy, and emotional regulation.

3. Continuous Education:

- **Advancement of Long lasting Learning**: Mental feeling and social commitment advance deep rooted learning and scholarly interest. Proceeding to master new abilities, investigate groundbreaking thoughts, and draw in with assorted viewpoints over the course of life upholds mental imperativeness and versatility.

- **Variation to Aging:** As people age, keeping up with mental and social commitment turns out to be progressively significant for saving mental capability and personal satisfaction. Remaining intellectually dynamic and socially associated can assist more seasoned grown-ups with adjusting to progress in years related changes and keep a feeling of direction and satisfaction.

In synopsis, mental feeling and social commitment are fundamental for keeping up with mental capability, advancing mind wellbeing, and improving general prosperity across life expectancy. By focusing on exercises that challenge the psyche and encourage social associations, people can uphold mental strength, diminish the gamble of mental deterioration, and partake in a better life.

Chapter 3

Diet and Nutrition

guidelines for a brain-healthy diet,

1. Foods grown from the ground

- Mean to remember various vivid products of the soil for your eating regimen, as various varieties demonstrate various phytochemicals and cancer prevention agents that advantage mind wellbeing.

- Choose leafy greens like Swiss chard, spinach, and kale, which are full of antioxidants, vitamins, and minerals.

- Consolidate berries like blueberries, strawberries, and raspberries, which are high in cancer prevention agents and have been connected to worked on mental capability.

- Incorporate other beautiful leafy foods like oranges, carrots, tomatoes, and ringer peppers, which give nutrients, fiber, and other gainful supplements.

2. Whole Grains:

Whenever possible, go with whole grains over refined ones because they have more fiber, vitamins, and minerals that are good for the brain.

- Incorporate entire grains like earthy colored rice, quinoa, oats, grain, and entire wheat in your eating routine.
- Limit admission of handled grains and refined starches, like white bread, white rice, and sweet oats, which can prompt spikes in glucose levels and aggravation.

3. Solid Fats:

- Remember wellsprings of solid fats for your eating regimen, like greasy fish, nuts, seeds, avocados, and olive oil.
- Greasy fish like salmon, mackerel, trout, and sardines are wealthy in omega-3 unsaturated fats, which are fundamental for mind wellbeing and mental capability.
- Nuts and seeds like flaxseeds, chia seeds, walnuts, almonds, and omega-3 fatty acids are good sources of fiber and antioxidants.
- Utilize olive oil as your essential cooking oil and salad dressing, as it is wealthy in monounsaturated fats and has calming properties.

4. Other Cerebrum Supporting Foods:

- Remember wellsprings of lean protein for your eating regimen, like poultry, eggs, vegetables, and tofu, which give amino acids fundamental for synapse amalgamation and mind capability.
- Consume moderate measures of dairy items, for example, yogurt and cheddar, which give calcium, vitamin D, and probiotics that help mind and stomach wellbeing.
- Limit admission of handled and sweet food sources, as over the top sugar utilization has been connected to irritation, oxidative pressure, and mental deterioration.

5. Hydration:

- Remain hydrated by drinking a lot of water over the course of the day, as drying out can debilitate mental capability and mind-set.

- Limit admission of sweet refreshments and energized drinks, as they can disturb hydration and lead to energy crashes.

By observing these rules and integrating cerebrum good food varieties into your eating routine, you can uphold mental capability, decrease the gamble of mental deterioration, and advance generally speaking mind wellbeing. Moreover, keeping a reasonable eating routine close by other way of life factors like customary activity, satisfactory rest, and stress the executives can additionally upgrade cerebrum wellbeing and prosperity.

- **The effect that particular dietary patterns and nutrients have on cognitive function.**

Explicit supplements and dietary examples assume vital parts in supporting mental capability and mind wellbeing. Here is a conversation of their effect:

1. Omega-3 Greasy Acids:

- Impact: Omega-3 unsaturated fats, especially EPA (eicosapentaenoic corrosive) and DHA (docosahexaenoic corrosive), are fundamental for cerebrum wellbeing. They play important roles in neurotransmission, synaptic plasticity, and inflammation regulation as structural brain cell membrane components.

- Sources: Greasy fish like salmon, mackerel, and sardines are rich wellsprings of EPA and DHA. Plant-based sources incorporate flaxseeds, chia seeds, pecans, and green growth based supplements.

Benefits: Utilization of omega-3 unsaturated fats has been related with worked on mental capability, memory, and state of mind. They may likewise diminish the gamble of mental degradation and dementia.

2. Antioxidants:

- Impact: Cancer prevention agents, including nutrients C and E, beta-carotene, and flavonoids, assist with safeguarding synapses from oxidative pressure and aggravation. Free radicals, which can harm brain cells and cause cognitive decline, are neutralized by them.

- Sources: Products of the soil are rich wellsprings of cell reinforcements, especially brilliant assortments, for example, berries, citrus organic products, salad greens, and cruciferous vegetables. Different sources incorporate nuts, seeds, entire grains, and flavors like turmeric.

- Benefits: Slims down high in cell reinforcements have been related with worked on mental capability, memory, and leader capability. They may likewise lessen the gamble old enough related mental deterioration and neurodegenerative infections.

3. Vitamin B12:

- Impact: B nutrients, including folate, vitamin B6, and vitamin B12, assume significant parts in synapse union, methylation processes, and homocysteine digestion. Cognitive impairment and neurodegenerative diseases have been linked to vitamin deficiencies.

- References: Wellsprings of folate incorporate mixed greens, vegetables, braced grains, and citrus natural products. Vitamin B6 is tracked down in poultry, fish, potatoes, and bananas, while vitamin B12 is principally found in creature items like meat, fish, dairy, and eggs.

Benefits: Satisfactory admission of B nutrients upholds mental capability, memory, and mind-set. Folate, specifically, has been related with a diminished gamble of mental degradation and Alzheimer's illness.

4. Mediterranean Diet:

- Impact: The Mediterranean eating regimen is wealthy in natural products, vegetables, entire grains, nuts, seeds, olive oil, and greasy fish, and low in red meat and handled food varieties. It gives an equilibrium between supplements and cell reinforcements that help mind wellbeing and diminish irritation.
- Advantages: Adherence to the Mediterranean eating regimen has been related with worked on mental capability, memory, and leader capability. Additionally,

it may lower the risk of neurodegenerative diseases like Alzheimer's and cognitive decline.

In conclusion, certain nutrients and dietary habits may have significant effects on brain health and cognitive function. Consolidating food sources plentiful in omega-3 unsaturated fats, cell reinforcements, B nutrients, and following a reasonable eating regimen, for example, the Mediterranean eating regimen can uphold mental capability, memory, and state of mind, and lessen the gamble of mental deterioration and neurodegenerative illnesses.

- **Reasonable methods for integrating smart dieting propensities into day to day existence.**

The following are some helpful hints for incorporating healthy eating habits into everyday life:

1. Prepare and Plan Meals:

- Prepare of time to guarantee you have nutritious choices accessible.
- Clump cook and plan dinners ahead of time to save time during occupied work days.
- Stock your storage room and cooler with solid staples like entire grains, lean proteins,

organic products, vegetables, nuts, and seeds.

2. Center around Entire Foods:

- Pick entire, insignificantly handled food sources over bundled and handled choices.
- Focus on foods grown from the ground as the underpinning of your feasts, intending to fill a portion of your plate with produce.
- Instead of refined grains, choose whole grains like brown rice, quinoa, oats, and whole wheat bread.

3. Segment Control:
- Focus on segment sizes to abstain from gorging, particularly with calorie-thick food varieties.
- Utilize more modest plates and bowls to assist with controlling part estimates and stay away from larger than usual servings.
- Be aware of piece sizes while eating out, as café segments will generally be bigger than needed.

4. Incorporate Protein at Each Meal:

- Integrate lean protein sources like poultry, fish, tofu, beans, lentils, and Greek yogurt into your feasts.
Protein supports muscle health, stabilizes blood sugar levels, and helps you feel full and satisfied.

5. Nibble Smart:

- Pick supplement thick tidbits, for example, new natural product, vegetables with hummus or nut margarine, Greek yogurt, nuts, seeds, or entire grain wafers.
By portioning out snacks ahead of time and storing them in single-serving containers, you can avoid mindless snacking.

6. Remain Hydrated:

- Drink a lot of water over the course of the day to remain hydrated and support generally wellbeing.

- Limit sweet refreshments and juiced drinks, as they can add to drying out and energy crashes.

7. Practice Careful Eating:
Eat slowly and mindfully, listening to your body's signals of hunger and fullness.
- Keep away from interruptions like TV or screens while eating, and appreciate each nibble.
- Tune into your body's signs of appetite and satiety, halting when you feel fulfilled instead of excessively full.

8. Consider Treats in Moderation:
Rather than completely depriving yourself, occasionally indulge in your favorite treats.
- Engage in mindful indulgence, savoring each bite without feeling guilty.

9. Be Adaptable and Forgiving:
- Embrace adaptability in your dietary patterns and consider periodic deviations from your standard daily schedule.

- Be pardoning of yourself assuming you get sidetracked sometimes, and center around pursuing better decisions in the long haul.

10. Look for Help and Accountability:
- Encircle yourself with strong companions, family, or networks who share your wellbeing objectives.
A registered dietitian or nutritionist can provide you with individualized guidance and hold you accountable.

By integrating these useful hints into your everyday daily schedule, you can lay out smart dieting propensities that help your general wellbeing and prosperity. Recall that little, reasonable changes after some time can prompt critical upgrades in your eating routine and in general wellbeing.

Chapter 4

Physical Activity and Exercise

The advantages of normal active work for mind wellbeing.

Customary active work offers various advantages for mind wellbeing, adding to worked on mental capability, temperament guideline, and generally prosperity. Here are a portion of the key advantages:

1. Expanded Blood Stream to the Brain: Practice increments blood stream to the

mind, conveying oxygen and supplements fundamental for ideal cerebrum capability. This improved blood stream advances neurogenesis (the development of new synapses) and brain adaptability (the cerebrum's capacity to adjust and redesign), which backing learning, memory, and mental capability.

2. Synapse Regulation: Active work animates the arrival of synapses like dopamine, serotonin, and norepinephrine, which assume key parts in mind-set guideline, stress decrease, and mental capability. These synapses advance sensations of joy, unwinding, and readiness, and assist with further developing concentration, consideration, and memory.

3. Cerebrum Inferred Neurotrophic Element (BDNF) Production: Practice expands the creation of cerebrum determined neurotrophic factor (BDNF), a protein that upholds the development,

endurance, and support of synapses. BDNF advances brain adaptability and synaptic pliancy, reinforcing brain associations and improving mental capability.

4. Reduction of Oxidative Stress and Inflammation: Standard actual work has calming and cancer prevention agent impacts, diminishing aggravation and oxidative pressure in the cerebrum. Constant irritation and oxidative pressure are embroiled in neurodegenerative sicknesses like Alzheimer's illness and Parkinson's illness, so decreasing these variables can help safeguard against mental deterioration and neurodegeneration.

5. Further developed Temperament and Stress Reduction: Endorphins and other "feel-good" chemicals are released during exercise, which improves mood and reduces stress, anxiety, and depression. Actual work additionally advances unwinding, further develops rest quality, and lifts confidence,

all of which add to better psychological wellness and prosperity.

6.   Improved Mental Capability and Scholastic Performance: Normal active work is related with worked on mental capability, including better memory, consideration, handling velocity, and leader capability. Kids and young people who participate in normal actual work might encounter improved scholastic execution and mental turn of events, as exercise animates mind districts engaged with learning and memory.

7. Decreased Chance of Mental degradation and Dementia: Various examinations have shown that standard active work is related with a diminished gamble of mental degradation and dementia in more established grown-ups. Practice advances cerebrum wellbeing all through the life expectancy, expanding mental save and diminishing the gamble old enough related

mental debilitation and neurodegenerative infections.

In conclusion, engaging in regular physical activity has a number of positive effects on brain health, including increased blood flow to the brain, regulation of neurotransmitters, production of BDNF, decreased inflammation and oxidative stress, improved mood and stress reduction, improved cognitive function and academic performance, and a lower risk of dementia and cognitive decline. Integrating normal activity into your routine is a strong method for supporting cerebrum wellbeing and generally speaking prosperity at whatever stage in life.

- **proposals for various kinds of activities and their effect on mental capability**

1. Vigorous Exercise:

- Recommendation: Aim for 75 minutes of vigorous-intensity aerobic exercise or 150 minutes of moderate-intensity aerobic exercise over several days each week. Models incorporate energetic strolling, running, cycling, swimming, moving, and high impact exercise classes.

-Influence on Mental Function: High-impact practice has been displayed to work on mental capability, including consideration, memory, handling rate, and chief capability. It increments blood stream to the cerebrum, advances the arrival of synapses like dopamine and serotonin, and animates the development of mind determined neurotrophic factor (BDNF), all of which backing cerebrum wellbeing and mental capability.

2. Strength Training:

- Recommendation: Integrate strength preparing practices somewhere around two days of the week, focusing on significant muscle gatherings like the legs, arms, back, chest, and center. Bodyweight exercises like squats, lunges, and push-ups, resistance band exercises, and using weight machines are all examples.

- Influence on Mental Function: While strength preparing principally centers around developing muscle fortitude and perseverance, it likewise has mental advantages. Research recommends that strength preparing can work on mental capability, especially chief capability and memory. It might likewise improve brain adaptability and advance the development of new synapses.

3. Adaptability and Equilibrium Exercises:

- Suggestions: Incorporate adaptability and equilibrium practices in your daily schedule something like a few times each week. Models incorporate yoga, jujitsu, Pilates, extending activities, and equilibrium preparing drills.
- Influence on Mental Function: Adaptability and equilibrium practices assist with keeping up with versatility, strength, and coordination, which are significant for by and large utilitarian freedom and personal satisfaction. While these activities may not straightforwardly influence mental capability, they add to by and large actual wellbeing and prosperity, which by implication upholds mind wellbeing.

4. Stop and go aerobic exercise (HIIT):

- Recommendation: Consolidate extreme cardio exercise (HIIT) into your normal one to two times each week, switching back and forth between short eruptions of serious activity and times of rest or lower-power movement. Sprint intervals, cycling sprints, and circuit training are examples.
- Influence on Mental Function: HIIT has been displayed to work on mental capability, memory, and leader capability, possibly more so than consistent state vigorous activity. It may support brain health and cognitive function by increasing levels of brain-derived neurotrophic factor (BDNF), promoting cardiovascular health, and enhancing neuroplasticity.

5. Mind-Body Exercises:

- Suggestions: Integrate mind-body activities like yoga, kendo, and qigong into your routine consistently, going for the gold a few meetings each week. These activities join actual development with care and breathwork.

- Influence on Mental Function: Mind-body practices have been related with worked on mental capability, consideration, and stress decrease. They advance unwinding, increment mindfulness, and upgrade mind-body association, which can decidedly affect cerebrum wellbeing and mental capability.

In outline, integrating various activities into your daily practice, including vigorous activity, strength preparing, adaptability and equilibrium works out, stop and go aerobic exercise (HIIT), and mind-body works out, can have critical advantages for mental capability and cerebrum wellbeing. To promote overall physical and mental health, take a diversified approach that incorporates a variety of exercises.

- **ways to incorporate exercise into daily routines for people of all ages and fitness levels.**

Regardless of age or fitness level, the following methods can be used to incorporate exercise into daily routines:

1. Begin Little and Slowly Increment Intensity:

- Start with short episodes of activity and step by step increment the length and force after some time as your wellness gets to the next level. Indeed, even only a couple of moments of movement can give medical advantages.
- Separate activity into more modest meetings over the course of the day if necessary. For instance, go for a 10-minute

stroll in the first part of the day, evening, and night.

2. Track down Exercises You Enjoy:

- Pick exercises that you appreciate and anticipate, whether it's strolling, swimming, moving, cultivating, or playing a game. Pleasant exercises are bound to turn into a normal piece of your everyday practice.
- Explore different avenues regarding various kinds of activity to find what turns out best for you. Keeping things interesting and avoiding boredom can be aided by variety.

3. Integrate Exercise into Everyday Tasks:

- Throughout the day, look for opportunities to exercise, such as taking the stairs rather than the elevator, parking further away from your destination, or running short errands by walking or biking.

- Transform family errands into potential open doors for development, for example, vacuuming, planting, or washing the vehicle. These exercises can consume calories and add to your everyday work-out objectives.

4. Set attainable objectives and monitor progress:

- Establish exercise objectives that are specific, attainable, and tailored to your fitness level and lifestyle. Begin with little, reasonable objectives and step by step increment the test after some time.
- Monitor your advancement to remain persuaded and praise your accomplishments. Utilize a wellness tracker, diary, or cell phone application to screen your movement levels and set updates for exercises.

5. Make Exercise a Priority:
- Plan practice into your day to day daily schedule as you would some other

significant arrangement or responsibility. Shut out time on your schedule for exercises and treat it as non-debatable.

- Focus on consistency over power. Try to get active every day, even if you can't do a full workout, to keep going and form new habits.

6. Amigo Up and Get Support:

- Practice with a companion, relative, or gathering to make it more pleasant and responsible. Having an exercise pal can give inspiration, backing, and brotherhood.

- To meet new people and stay motivated, join a walking group, sports team, or fitness class. Bunch exercise can add a social component to exercises and make them more pleasant.

7. Be Adaptable and Adjust to Changes:

- Your exercise routine should be adaptable and flexible, especially during busy or

challenging times. Acknowledge that there might be difficulties or snags, and spotlight on tracking down clever fixes to remain dynamic.
- Adjust exercises as necessary to accommodate any health issues or physical limitations. Talk with a medical care proficient or health specialist for customized direction and changes.

By integrating these procedures into your day to day daily practice, you can make practice a normal and charming piece of your way of life, paying little mind to mature or wellness level. Recall that each and every piece of movement counts, and, surprisingly, little changes can prompt huge enhancements in wellbeing and prosperity after some time.

Chapter 5

Mental Stimulation and Brain Training

significance of mental commitment and deep rooted learning. Mental commitment and long lasting learning are fundamental parts of keeping up with mind wellbeing, mental capability, and in general prosperity over the course of life.

Here's the reason they are significant:

1. Neurogenesis and plasticity of the brain:
- Mental commitment and deep rooted learning advance cerebrum pliancy, the

mind's capacity to adjust, redesign, and structure new associations because of encounters and boosts. Constant learning animates brain movement and supports neurogenesis, the development of new synapses, which are critical for mental capability and strength.

2. Mental Reserve: Cognitive reserve, a type of brain resilience that enables individuals to better withstand age-related changes and pathology, is built through intellectually stimulating activities. Mental save goes about as a support against mental degradation and neurodegenerative infections, permitting people to keep up with mental capability and freedom for longer periods.

3. Memory and Mental Function: - Mental commitment and long lasting learning challenge the mind, further develop memory, and upgrade different mental capabilities, for example, consideration, critical thinking, decisive reasoning, and independent direction. Mastering new abilities, dialects, or ideas fortifies brain associations and improves mental adaptability and effectiveness.

4. Mind-set and Profound Well-being:
- Long lasting learning and mental commitment add to profound prosperity and mental flexibility. They offer chances for intellectual stimulation, creative expression, and personal development, which can help people feel better about themselves, have more confidence, and have a sense of purpose. Besides reducing stress, anxiety, and depression, engaging in meaningful activities and pursuing interests can also help.

5. Social Cooperation and Connection:
- Long lasting advancing frequently includes social communication and association with other people who share comparable interests and interests. Partaking in classes,

studios, conversation gatherings, or local area exercises cultivates social commitment, assembles interpersonal organizations, and improves social help, which are significant for in general prosperity and personal satisfaction.

6. Adaptation to Changes in Life:

- Deep rooted learning works with transformation to life changes and difficulties by giving open doors to individual and scholarly development. Whether exploring profession changes, retirement, feeling of emptiness after the last kid left home, or other life advances, mastering new abilities, investigating new interests, and remaining mentally drawn in can advance versatility and an uplifting perspective on life.

7. Upgraded Nature of Life:

- Deep rooted learning enhances valuable encounters, widens points of view, and cultivates a feeling of interest, miracle, and satisfaction. It energizes investigation, disclosure, and deep rooted interest on the planet, prompting a more significant and intentional presence. In conclusion, lifelong learning and cognitive engagement are essential for preserving brain health, cognitive function, and emotional well-being throughout one's lifetime.

By embracing scholarly excitement, seeking after interests, and ceaselessly testing the brain, people can upgrade mental hold, versatility, and personal satisfaction, empowering them to flourish notwithstanding life's difficulties and changes.

- **instances of exercises that animate the mind and advance mental commitment:**

1. Brainteasers and Puzzles: -

Puzzles to stimulate your brain

Word search

S E A S T E R R C H I C
C E E E A G O A A N T A
S H H C M G A A R C R G
F P O C O S O C R L A R
B T P C F I R T O E B A
U H S H O I S T T R B N
N E E E E L V A P R I L
N R N T V N A X N T T M
Y V B A S K E T C H R A
P P I E O S N S E E R H
A H O L I D A Y G R R E
S H U S T H T E H U N T

HOP	CHIC	EASTER	CHOCOLATE
HUNT	RABBIT	BASKET	HOLIDAY
EGGS	APRIL	BUNNY	CARROT

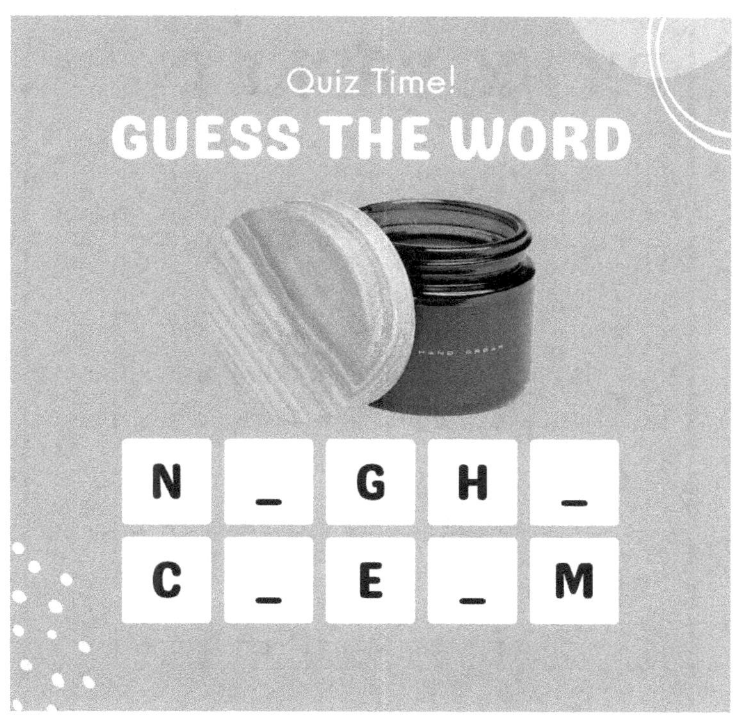

Quiz Time!
GUESS THE WORD
N _ G H _
C _ E _ M

PICNIC BASKET

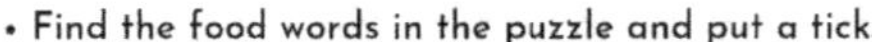

• Find the food words in the puzzle and put a tick.

w	a	t	e	r	m	e	l	o	n
d	b	l	e	m	o	n	a	d	e
b	a	p	p	l	e	d	l	t	q
u	n	n	g	r	a	p	e	s	g
r	a	i	c	o	t	h	p	x	e
g	n	d	a	w	c	h	i	p	s
e	a	r	k	s	i	p	a	m	m
r	s	h	e	c	t	s	u	k	i
m	s	a	n	d	w	i	c	h	l
c	o	o	k	i	e	s	s	e	k
c	h	o	c	o	l	a	t	e	d

1. 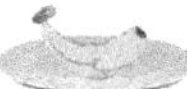 2. 3. 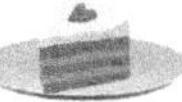 4.

5. 6. 7. 8.

9. 10. 11.

2.Games and Challenges:
  - Prepackaged games (e.g., Scrabble, Chess, Pilgrims of Catan)
  - Card games like solitaire, bridge, and poker
  - Methodology games (e.g., Hazard, Stratego, Human progress)
  - Quiz games
  - Memory games (e.g., Fixation, Memory Match)

3. Learning and Reading:

  - Understanding books, papers, magazines, and online articles
  - acquiring new language skills

- Taking classes or studios on different subjects (e.g., workmanship, history, science)
- Paying attention to instructive digital broadcasts or book recordings
- Investigating on the web courses or instructional exercises (e.g., Coursera, Khan Institute, TED-Ed)

4. Imaginative Activities:
- Composing (e.g., journaling, exploratory writing, verse)
- Drawing, painting, or different types of creative articulation
- Making (e.g., weaving, sewing, carpentry)
- Playing an instrument or creating music

5. Critical thinking and Basic Thinking:
-Participating in discussions or conversations on different subjects
- Addressing real-world challenges or issues
- Partaking in get away from rooms or secret tackling exercises

- Dissecting and deciphering information or data

- Exploring different avenues regarding groundbreaking thoughts or creations

6.Proactive tasks with Mental Components: - Moving (which includes remembering steps, arrangements, and examples)

- Combative techniques (which requires concentration, procedure, and coordination) - Yoga or kendo (which consolidates actual development with care and fixation)

- Open air exercises like climbing, orienteering, or geocaching (which include route and critical thinking)

7. Innovation Based Mind Training: - Utilizing cerebrum preparing applications or programming intended to work on mental abilities (e.g., Lumosity, Raise, Pinnacle)

- Playing instructive computer games or reproductions that challenge mental capacities (e.g., Entryway, The Observer, Progress)

By integrating these exercises into your everyday practice, you can invigorate your mind, improve mental capability, and advance deep rooted learning and mental dexterity.

Assortment is critical, so attempt to take part in a blend of exercises that challenge different mental abilities and interests.

- **Methodologies for keeping up with mental spryness and testing the psyche.**

Strategies for challenging one's mind and maintaining mental agility include the following:

1. Participate in Lifelong Education:
- Take classes, studios, or courses on subjects that interest you. Investigate new

subjects and subject matters to keep your brain drew in and animated.

- Go to talks, talks, or online courses on recent developments, science, history, or different subjects to remain informed and mentally locked in.

- Sign up for online courses or instructive stages that offer many subjects and learning valuable open doors.

2. Seek after Scholarly Hobbies:

- Participate in leisure activities that require mental exertion and critical thinking, like riddles, games, and puzzles. - Investigate innovative pursuits like composition, drawing, painting, or creating, which invigorate the creative mind and mental abilities. - Become familiar with an instrument, work on singing, or form music to challenge hear-able and coordinated movements while cultivating innovativeness.

3. Peruse Broadly and Critically:

- Understand books, papers, magazines, and online articles on assorted subjects to grow your insight and viewpoints.

- Examine and scrutinize the data you experience, taking into account various perspectives and assessing sources basically.
- Join a book club or conversation gathering to take part in discussions about writing, thoughts, and recent developments.

4. Maintain intellectual and social engagement:

- Keep up with social associations with companions, family, and friends through standard discussions, trips, or gathering exercises.

- Partake in conversations, discussions, or gatherings on subjects of interest, either face to face or on the web. Volunteer for causes or organizations that align with your values and interests, which will give you chances to meet new people and stimulate your mind.

5. Practice Care and Meditation:

- Consolidate care practices like reflection, profound breathing activities, or yoga into your day to day daily schedule to upgrade concentration, consideration, and close to home guideline.
- Practice careful familiarity with your viewpoints, sentiments, and sensations, developing a non-critical disposition and present-second mindfulness.

6. Challenge Yourself with New Experiences:

- Get out of your usual range of familiarity and attempt new exercises or encounters that stretch your capacities and points of view.
- Go to new spots, investigate various societies, and drench yourself in new conditions to animate interest and flexibility.
- Take on new obligations or jobs that require critical thinking, navigation, and acquiring new abilities.

7. Remain Truly Active:

- Customary actual work has been connected to worked on mental capability, memory, and mental spryness. Integrate practice into your daily schedule to help mind wellbeing and generally speaking prosperity.

- Pick exercises that challenge coordination, equilibrium, and coordinated abilities, like moving, combative techniques, or sports.

8. Maintain a well-balanced life:

- In order to support cognitive function and mental well-being, prioritize getting enough sleep, eating well, and managing stress. For stress reduction and mental clarity, try relaxing techniques like deep breathing, progressive muscle relaxation, or visualization.

- Look for proficient assistance on the off chance that you experience tireless emotional well-being concerns or mental hardships, as early mediation can prompt improved results.

By integrating these methodologies into your way of life, you can keep up with mental readiness, animate your brain, and advance deep rooted learning and mental essentialness. Embrace interest, challenge yourself routinely, and stay open to new encounters and open doors for development.

Daily Habit

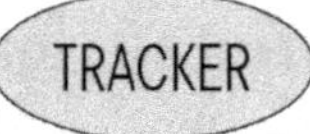

Manage your habits to stay focused and achieve your goals. Jot down your
top habits and track your progress each day as you accomplish them.

Meditate for 5 Minutes

S M T W T F S

Learn something new

S M T W T F S

Limit Social Media Use

S M T W T F S

Get 8 Hours of Sleep

S M T W T F S

New habit

TRACKER

Manage your habits to stay focused and achieve your goals. Jot down your
top habits and track your progress each day as you accomplish them.

Drink Enough Water

S M T W T F S

Read or listen to podcasts for 20 minutes

S M T W T F S

Exercise or 10 Minute Walk

S M T W T F S

Socialize

S M T W T F S

Chapter 6

Social Engagement and Relationships

Association between friendly associations and mental wellbeing.

Social associations assume a vital part in keeping up with mental wellbeing and by and large prosperity. This is the way friendly associations are associated with mental wellbeing:

1. Cognitive Function Stimulation: - Social collaborations give open doors to mental feeling and commitment. Discussions, discussions, and conversations with others challenge mental cycles like consideration, memory, language, and critical thinking, keeping the cerebrum dynamic and deft.

2. Consistent reassurance and Stress Reduction:

- Solid social associations offer close to home help and buffering against pressure. Having a steady organization of companions, family, and friends can assist people with adapting to life's difficulties and lessen sensations of tension, melancholy, and dejection, which can adversely influence mental capability.

3. Promoting the health of the brain:

- Social commitment has been connected to better mental capability and a diminished gamble of mental degradation and dementia. Collaborating with others animates mind districts engaged with social perception, sympathy, and close to home guideline, which are significant for keeping up with cerebrum wellbeing and versatility.

4. Improvement of Mental Well-being: Social connections enhance psychological resilience and mental well-being. Feeling associated with others cultivates a feeling of having a place, reason, and significance throughout everyday life, which are related with better mental capability and by and large personal satisfaction.

5. Mental Hold and Adaptability:
 - Social associations are one part of mental hold, a defensive element that empowers the mind to endure age-related changes and pathology. Having a rich informal organization and taking part in friendly exercises over the course of life add to mental hold, improving the mind's flexibility and versatility to mental degradation.

6. Opportunities for Continuing Education:

- Social collaborations frequently include sharing information, encounters, and viewpoints with others. Taking part in discussions, bunch exercises, and cooperative activities gives amazing open doors to deep rooted learning, scholarly feeling, and mental development.

7. Actual Wellbeing Benefits:

- Better physical health outcomes, including lower rates of chronic diseases like heart disease, diabetes, and hypertension, have been linked to strong social connections. For preserving cognitive function and lowering the likelihood of cognitive decline, it is essential to maintain good physical health.

In a nutshell, opportunities for lifelong learning, mental stimulation, emotional support, stress relief, and social connections are all intertwined with cognitive health. By sustaining social connections and remaining associated with others, people can uphold their mental capability, advance mind wellbeing, and upgrade in general prosperity over the course of life.

- advantages of keeping up with companionships, taking part in bunch exercises, and drawing in with local area associations.

There are numerous advantages to maintaining friendships, participating in group activities, and getting involved with community organizations for mental, emotional, and physical health. Here are a portion of the key advantages:

1. Social Help and Profound Well-being: Emotional support, companionship, and a sense of belonging are all provided by friendships. Having dear companions to trust in and share encounters with can diminish sensations of depression, stress, and uneasiness, advancing profound prosperity and flexibility.

2. Stress Decrease and Adapting Mechanisms:

- Investing energy with companions and participating in agreeable gathering exercises can act as successful pressure supports. Social help from companions and friends can assist people with adapting to life's difficulties, giving solace, point of view, and useful help when required.

3. Improved Mental Spryness and Mental Function:

- Social communications and gathering exercises animate mental capability, testing the cerebrum and keeping it light-footed. Taking part in discussions, discusses, and cooperative tasks with others gives potential open doors to scholarly feeling, critical thinking, and realizing, which can upgrade mental capability and versatility.

4. Promoting physical health and happiness:

- Taking part in bunch exercises and local area associations frequently includes actual development and exercise, which adds to better actual wellbeing results. Walking, dancing, or playing sports with friends are all forms of regular physical activity that support cardiovascular health, muscle strength, and overall well-being.

5. Feeling of Direction and Significant Connections:

- Contribution in local area associations and gathering exercises encourages a feeling of direction and association with an option that could be bigger than oneself. Pursuing shared objectives, chipping in for purposes you trust in, and adding to the prosperity of others can give a feeling of satisfaction and importance throughout everyday life.

6. Development of Informal communities and Social Skills:

- Taking part in bunch exercises and local area associations opens people to different points of view, societies, and foundations, growing their informal communities and interactive abilities. Associating with individuals from various different backgrounds cultivates sympathy, understanding, and social capability, upgrading relational connections and relational abilities.

7. Long lasting Learning and Individual Growth:

- Bunch exercises and local area contribution give valuable open doors to deep rooted learning, expertise advancement, and self-awareness. Engaging in activities with other people, such as attending workshops, joining clubs, or taking part in community events, encourages ongoing learning and self-improvement by promoting intellectual curiosity, creativity, and curiosity about one's own mind.

8. Decrease of Social Disengagement and Loneliness:

- Partaking in bunch exercises and keeping up with fellowships helps battle social disengagement and depression, especially among more established grown-ups or people who might be in danger of feeling detached. The quality of one's life as a whole can be improved by establishing and maintaining social connections.

In synopsis, keeping up with kinships, taking part in bunch exercises, and drawing in with local area associations offer a large number of advantages for mental, close to home, and actual prosperity. By sustaining social connections, remaining dynamic in social environments, and adding to local area life, people can improve their social encouraging groups of people, advance mental capability, and lead satisfying and significant lives. ways to encourage social associations and building significant connections.

- **few ways to cultivate social associations and building significant connections**:

1. Be Open and Approachable:

- Move toward social circumstances with a receptive outlook and a cordial disposition. Grin, visually connect, and start discussions with others in an inviting way.
- Be responsive to meeting new individuals and shaping associations, regardless of whether it feels awkward from the start.

2. Be Genuinely Involved in Others

- Get clarification on pressing issues and effectively pay attention to others while taking part in discussion. Show certifiable interest in their inclinations, encounters, and points of view.

- Show compassion and grasping by approving others' sentiments and encounters, regardless of whether they vary from your own.

3. Be True and Vulnerable:

- Authentically share your own thoughts, emotions, and experiences with others. Show weakness and offer both the ups and downs of your life. Because it allows for genuine and meaningful interactions, authenticity fosters trust and deeper connections with others.

4. Track down Normal Interests and Activities:

- Search out chances to interface with other people who share comparative interests, leisure activities, or interests. Join clubs, classes, or gatherings zeroed in on exercises you appreciate.

- Take part in bunch exercises, group activities, or volunteer undertakings where you can team up with others towards shared objectives.

5. Remain Associated and Connect Regularly:

- Keep in touch with companions, family, and colleagues by booking time to associate, whether it's through calls, video talks, or in-person gatherings.

- Really try to contact others, particularly during testing times or times of progress. Offer help, support, and a listening ear when required.

6. Be Available and Taken part in Relationships:

- Be completely present and mindful while investing energy with others. Set aside interruptions, for example, telephones or electronic gadgets and spotlight on the individual you're collaborating with.

- Practice undivided attention and answer nicely to what others are talking about, exhibiting sympathy and understanding.

7. Develop Significant Associations Over Quantity:

- Center around developing a couple of close, significant connections instead of attempting to keep an enormous organization of shallow associations.
- Put time and exertion into sustaining these connections, focusing on quality communications and close to home closeness.

8. Express Your Appreciation and Gratitude:

- Show appreciation for individuals in your day to day existence by offering thanks for their presence, backing, and commitments.
- Send manually written notes, messages, or messages communicating thanks and telling others you esteem their kinship and friendship.

9. Be Patient and Understanding:

- Comprehend that building significant connections requires some investment and exertion. Be patient and give connections the space to foster normally over the long haul.
- Be comprehension of others' disparities, characteristics, and limits, and regard their independence and independence.

10. Look for Proficient Assistance When Needed:

- On the off chance that you're battling to frame significant associations or keep up with connections because of fundamental issues like social nervousness or discouragement, think about looking for help from a specialist or instructor.
- Proficient direction can assist you with creating survival methods, further develop relational abilities, and explore relational difficulties all the more successfully.

By carrying out these tips into your day to day routine, you can encourage social associations, construct significant connections, and develop a strong organization of companions, family, and friends. Recall that certifiable associations require some investment and exertion, however the prizes of significant connections are definitely justified.

Chapter 7

Sleep and Stress Management

significance of value rest for mind wellbeing and mental capability. Sleeping well is important for the brain's health and ability to think clearly. This is why:

1. Memory Consolidation: During rest, the mind merges recollections and cycles data from the day. This interaction is essential for learning and holding new data, as well concerning making associations between various snippets of data.

2. Cerebrum Plasticity: Rest assumes a key part in mind versatility, the mind's capacity to adjust and rearrange itself in light of new encounters and learning. Satisfactory rest upholds synaptic pliancy, the reinforcing and development of associations between neurons, which is fundamental for mental capability and learning.

3. Attention and Concentration: Getting enough sleep improves cognitive performance as well as attention and concentration. Lack of sleep can impede mental capability, prompting troubles with memory, critical thinking, direction, and response times.

4. Emotional Regulation: Getting enough sleep is essential for maintaining a stable mood and emotional balance. Satisfactory rest controls feelings, decrease pressure, and advance mental prosperity. Lack of sleep, then again, can prompt crabbiness, state of mind swings, and expanded vulnerability to stress and uneasiness.

5. Clearing Cerebrum Toxins: During rest, the mind gets out poisons and byproducts that amass during waking hours. This interaction, known as the glymphatic framework, keeps up with cerebrum wellbeing and may decrease the gamble of neurodegenerative illnesses like Alzheimer's sickness.

6. Ideal Cerebrum Function: Quality rest upholds ideal mind capability across different mental spaces, including consideration, memory, critical thinking, innovativeness, and independent direction. Reliably getting sufficient top notch rest is fundamental for keeping up with mental execution and generally speaking cerebrum wellbeing.

7. Cerebrum Wellbeing and Longevity: Constant lack of sleep has been related with an expanded gamble of mental degradation, neurodegenerative infections, and other neurological issues. Focusing on quality rest over the course of life might help safeguard against age-related mental deterioration and advance cerebrum wellbeing and life span.

In outline, quality rest is fundamental for cerebrum wellbeing and mental capability. It upholds memory union, mind versatility, consideration, focus, profound guideline, poison leeway, ideal cerebrum capability, and may decrease the gamble of mental degradation and neurodegenerative sicknesses.

Focusing on solid rest propensities and guaranteeing sufficient rest is fundamental for by and large mental execution and prosperity.

- **Techniques for further developing rest cleanliness and tending to normal rest issues.**

Here are techniques for further developing rest cleanliness and tending to normal rest issues:

1. Lay out a Reliable Rest Schedule:

- Set a regular time for going to bed and waking up each day, even on weekends. Consistency directs your body's inner clock and further develops rest quality.

2. Make a Loosening up Sleep time Routine:

- Foster a quieting sleep time routine to indicate to your body that now is the ideal time to slow down. This might incorporate exercises like perusing, washing up, rehearsing unwinding strategies, or paying attention to relieving music.

3. Enhance Your Sleeping Space:

- Make the environment conducive to sleep comfortable. Invest in a supportive mattress and pillows to keep your bedroom cool, quiet, and dark. Reduce the amount of noise and other sources of distraction, such as bright lights, electronic devices, or loud noises, that could disrupt your sleep.

4. Limit screen time before bedtime:

- Try not to utilize electronic gadgets, for example, cell phones, tablets, PCs, and televisions in the hour paving the way to sleep time. The blue light radiated by screens can stifle melatonin creation and obstruct rest.

5. Screen Your Caffeine and Liquor Intake:

- Limit utilization of caffeine, nicotine, and liquor, particularly some time before sleep time. These substances can disturb rest designs and diminish rest quality.

6. Regular physical activity, but not too close to bedtime:

- Get active on a regular basis, but avoid intense activity right before bedtime because it may wake you up and disrupt your sleep. Expect to complete activity basically a couple of hours before sleep time.

7. Oversee Pressure and Anxiety:

- Practice pressure decreasing strategies like profound breathing, reflection, care, or moderate muscle unwinding to advance unwinding and ease uneasiness before sleep time.

- Think about keeping a concern diary to write down any worries or considerations before bed, permitting you to handle them and let them go.

8. Watch Your Eating routine and Hydration:

- Close to bedtime, avoid large meals, spicy foods, and a lot of liquids because they can make you feel uncomfortable and make it hard to sleep. Settle on a light tidbit on the off chance that you're eager before bed.

- Remain hydrated over the course of the day, however decrease liquid admission in the hours paving the way to sleep time to limit evening arousals for washroom trips.

9. Look for Proficient Assistance for Tenacious Rest Issues:

- In the event that you experience determined rest troubles or suspect you might have a rest problem like a sleeping disorder, rest apnea, fretful legs condition, or narcolepsy, look for assessment and treatment from a medical services proficient.

- A medical services supplier might suggest mental conduct treatment for sleep deprivation (CBT-I), medicine, or different mediations custom fitted to your particular rest needs.

10. Consistently practice good sleep hygiene:

- Focus on rest cleanliness and integrate these techniques into your day to day schedule reliably. Consistency is critical to further developing rest quality and laying out sound rest propensities over the long run. You can improve your sleep quality, duration, and overall well-being by implementing these methods for addressing common sleep disorders and improving your sleep hygiene.

Recollect that singular rest needs shift, so it's vital to find what turns out best for yourself and make changes depending on the situation.

- **procedures for overseeing pressure and advancing unwinding:**

1. Care Meditation:

- Practice care contemplation by concentrating on the current second without judgment. Sit discreetly, shut your eyes, and carry your attention to your breath, substantial sensations, or environmental elements.

- Notice any considerations, sentiments, or impressions that emerge, and essentially notice them without becoming involved with them. When your mind wanders, bring it back to the here and now.

- Begin with short meetings of 5-10 minutes and progressively increment the term as you become more alright with the training.

2. Profound Breathing Exercises:

- Practice profound breathing activities to quiet the psyche and body. Sit or rests in an agreeable position and take slow, full breaths through your nose, filling your lungs with air.

- Pause your breathing for a couple of moments, then breathe out leisurely through your mouth, delivering pressure and stress with every breath.

- Center around the beat of your breath, permitting it to turn out to be increasingly slow even with every inward breath and exhalation.

3. Progressive muscle relaxation (PMR):

- Practice moderate muscle unwinding to deliver pressure and advance unwinding all through your body. Begin by straining explicit muscle gatherings, like your clench hands, arms, shoulders, or legs, for a couple of moments.

- Then, gradually discharge the pressure and let the muscles unwind totally, seeing the distinction in sensation among strain and unwinding. Travel through each muscle bunch, working your direction from head to toe.

4. Body Sweep Meditation:

- Practice a body check reflection to carry attention to various pieces of your body and delivery pressure. Close your eyes and lie down in a comfortable position.

 - Start by zeroing in on your breath, then, at that point, step by step shift your consideration regarding various pieces of your body, beginning from your toes and moving vertical.

- Notice any areas of strain, inconvenience, or sensation as you examine each piece of your body, and permit them to unwind and relax with every breath.

5. Directed Symbolism and Visualization:

- Utilize directed symbolism and representation to make a psychological picture or situation that advances unwinding and tranquility. Shut your eyes and envision yourself in a quiet, tranquil setting, like an ocean side, backwoods, or peak.

- Picture the sights, sounds, and vibes of this serene spot, permitting yourself to completely submerge in the experience and let go of pressure and stresses.

6. Tai chi and yoga:

- Practice yoga or jujitsu to consolidate actual development with care and unwinding. Relaxation, flexibility, and mental clarity are all facilitated by these mind-body practices that include gentle stretching, meditation, and breathing exercises.

- Join a yoga or judo class, or track with online recordings or applications to learn and rehearse these strategies at home.

7. Nature Strolls and Outside Activities:

- Invest energy in nature and take part in outside exercises like strolling, climbing, or cultivating to advance unwinding and diminish pressure. Nature significantly affects the brain and body, assisting with reestablishing a feeling of equilibrium and prosperity.

 - Go for relaxed strolls in parks or normal regions, take in the outside air, and absorb the sights and hints of the regular world around you.

8. Journaling and Expressive Writing:

- Use journaling or expressive composition as a device for self-reflection, profound handling, and stress the board. Write about your experiences, feelings, and thoughts every day in a journal or notebook.

- Investigate your feelings, difficulties, and experiences through composition, permitting yourself to communicate and deliver repressed pressure or strain. By integrating these strategies into your everyday daily schedule, you can successfully oversee pressure, advance unwinding, and develop a more noteworthy feeling of smoothness and prosperity in your life.

Explore different avenues regarding various methods to find what turns out best for you, and practice routinely to receive the rewards of pressure decrease and unwinding.

Chapter 8

Managing Health Conditions

The effect of normal medical issue, like diabetes, hypertension, and corpulence, on mental capability. Normal medical issue like diabetes, hypertension, and weight can essentially affect mental capability.

This is the way each condition influences mental wellbeing:

1. Diabetes: - Diabetes, particularly when uncontrolled, can unfavorably affect mental capability. Constant high glucose levels can prompt aggravation, oxidative pressure, and harm to veins in the cerebrum, disabling mental cycles.

Diabetes increases a person's risk of developing vascular dementia, a type of dementia caused by damage to blood vessels that reduces blood flow to the brain.

- Diabetes is additionally connected with an expanded gamble of Alzheimer's illness and different types of dementia, potentially because of insulin obstruction and impeded glucose digestion in the cerebrum.

2. Hypertension (High Blood Pressure):

- Hypertension can harm veins all through the body, remembering those for the mind. Ongoing hypertension can prompt restricting and solidifying of veins, lessening blood stream to the mind and expanding the gamble of mental impedance.

- Hypertension is a huge gamble factor for vascular dementia, as it adds to the improvement of little vessel illness and white matter sores in the cerebrum, which are trademark elements of this kind of dementia.

- Uncontrolled hypertension is likewise connected with an expanded gamble of Alzheimer's infection and different types of dementia, conceivably through instruments connected with cerebral hypoperfusion, oxidative pressure, and aggravation.

3. Obesity:

- Heftiness is related with different metabolic and cardiovascular gamble factors that can adversely influence mental capability. Insulin resistance, dyslipidemia, inflammation, and oxidative stress are just a few of the conditions that can cause cognitive decline.

- Stoutness is connected to primary and utilitarian changes in the cerebrum, remembering adjustments for mind volume, white matter uprightness, and availability between mind areas. Memory, attention, and executive function may all be affected by these changes.

- Corpulence in midlife has been recognized as an endanger factor for dementia further down the road, especially Alzheimer's illness. The components hidden this affiliation might include insulin obstruction, dysregulation of adipokines (chemicals emitted by fat tissue), and persistent irritation. Generally, normal medical issue like diabetes, hypertension, and weight can significantly affect mental capability and increment the gamble of mental deterioration and dementia. Dealing with these circumstances through way of life adjustments (like solid eating regimen, customary activity, and weight the executives) and fitting clinical treatment is fundamental for protecting mental wellbeing and lessening the gamble of mental impedance. Also, checking and controlling other gamble factors like elevated cholesterol, smoking, and inactive way of life are significant for keeping up with ideal mind capability and by and large prosperity.

- **Direction for dealing with these circumstances through way of life changes, prescription, and standard medical services observing.**

Here's direction for overseeing normal ailments like diabetes, hypertension, and heftiness through way of life changes, drug, and ordinary medical care observing:

1. Diabetes:Way of life Changes:

- Follow a fair eating routine wealthy in natural products, vegetables, entire grains, lean proteins, and solid fats. Limit admission of sweet and high-carb food sources.

- Participate in standard actual work, holding back nothing 150 minutes of moderate-force vigorous activity each week, alongside muscle-fortifying exercises on at least two days of the week.

- Keep an eye on your blood sugar levels on a regular basis and follow your doctor's instructions for managing diabetes, such as taking insulin or other treatments.

Medication: - To keep your blood sugar levels under control and prevent complications related to diabetes, follow the instructions given to you by your doctor or other healthcare provider.   Depending on your specific requirements and current health status, you may be prescribed oral, injectable, or other diabetes medications.

Normal Medical care Monitoring:

- Go to customary check-ups with your medical care supplier to screen glucose levels, evaluate diabetes-related confusions, and change therapy plans depending on the situation.

- Plan customary eye tests, foot tests, and screenings for kidney capability, cholesterol levels, and cardiovascular wellbeing to screen for diabetes-related entanglements.

2. Hypertension (High Blood Pressure):Way of life Changes:

- Embrace a heart-solid eating routine, like the Scramble (Dietary Ways to deal with Stop Hypertension) diet, which underscores organic products, vegetables, entire grains, lean proteins, and low-fat dairy items while restricting sodium, immersed fats, and added sugars.

- Keep a sound load through a fair eating regimen and normal actual work. Even a modest weight loss can help lower blood pressure. Control your stress by practicing deep breathing, yoga, or other forms of relaxation, quitting smoking if necessary, and limiting your intake of alcohol.

Medication: - Take the medications your doctor has prescribed to lower your blood pressure and lower your risk of complications caused by hypertension. -

Antihypertensive meds like ACE inhibitors, angiotensin II receptor blockers (ARBs), diuretics, beta-blockers, and calcium channel blockers might be endorsed in view of your singular requirements and wellbeing status.

Normal Medical care Monitoring:

- Use a home blood pressure monitor to keep tabs on your blood pressure on a regular basis and report any readings to your doctor.

- Go to standard check-ups with your medical services supplier to screen pulse, survey cardiovascular wellbeing, and change therapy plans depending on the situation.

3. Obesity:Way of life Changes:

- Embrace a fair eating regimen that stresses entire, negligibly handled food varieties and incorporates various natural products, vegetables, lean proteins, and solid fats. Keep away from unnecessary admission of fatty, low-supplement food sources.   - Participate in customary actual work, holding back nothing 150 minutes of moderate-power vigorous activity each week, alongside muscle-fortifying exercises on at least two days of the week. - Put forth sensible objectives for weight reduction and spotlight on making manageable way of life changes, for example, segment control, careful eating, and customary activity. Medication: - At times, weight reduction meds might be endorsed by your medical care supplier to support weight the board, especially for people with heftiness related unexpected problems.

- These prescriptions work by smothering hunger, decreasing retention of supplements, or expanding digestion. They are not suitable for everyone and are typically used in conjunction with lifestyle changes.

Customary Medical services Monitoring: - Go to your doctor's office on a regular basis to have your weight, health, and progress toward your weight loss goals checked.

- Examine any difficulties or concerns you might have with weight the executives and work with your medical care supplier to change therapy plans on a case by case basis.

It is essential to collaborate closely with your healthcare provider to develop a bespoke treatment plan that is tailored to your specific requirements, health status, and lifestyle, in addition to these general guidelines. Customary observing, medicine adherence, and continuous help from medical services experts are fundamental for dealing with these circumstances really and lessening the gamble of entanglements.

Chapter 9

Preventive Measures and Risk Reduction

preventive measures for diminishing the gamble of dementia. Here are key preventive measures for lessening the gamble of dementia:

1. Maintain a healthy way of life:
   - Follow a reasonable eating routine wealthy in natural products, vegetables, entire grains, lean proteins, and solid fats. Limit admission of handled food varieties, sweet bites, and high-fat food varieties.
   - Participate in standard actual work, going for the gold 150 minutes of moderate-power

vigorous activity each week, alongside muscle-reinforcing exercises on at least two days out of every week.

- Try not to smoke and restrict liquor utilization to lessen the gamble of vascular and neurodegenerative sicknesses.

2. Manage and monitor persistent health conditions:

- Keep persistent ailments like diabetes, hypertension, and weight taken care of through way of life alterations, prescription adherence, and normal medical services checking.

- Work with your medical care supplier to foster a far reaching therapy plan customized to your singular necessities and wellbeing status.

3. Maintain intellectual and social engagement:

- Keep up with social associations with companions, family, and friends through ordinary cooperations, excursions, and gathering exercises.

- Participate in mentally animating exercises like perusing, puzzles, games, mastering new abilities, or taking classes to keep your cerebrum dynamic and locked in.

4. Focus on Quality Sleep: To promote restful and rejuvenating sleep, establish a regular sleep schedule and practice good sleep hygiene practices.

- Make a loosening up sleep time schedule, streamline your rest climate, and keep away from energizers like caffeine and electronic gadgets before sleep time.

5. Oversee Pressure and Mental Health: To promote emotional well-being and lower the likelihood of developing chronic stress, try stress-reduction methods like mindfulness, meditation, deep breathing exercises, and relaxation techniques.

- Look for help from medical services experts assuming you experience industrious psychological well-being concerns or troubles adapting to pressure.

6. Safeguard Your Head: - Wearing helmets while participating in sports and adhering to safety guidelines at work and at home are two ways to reduce the risk of traumatic brain injury and prevent head injuries.

7. Heed Clinical Guidance and Screening Recommendations:
- Go to customary check-ups with your medical services supplier to screen generally speaking wellbeing, survey mental capability, and examine any worries or changes in memory or thinking.
- Heed clinical guidance and evaluating proposals for early recognition and the executives of conditions that might build the gamble of dementia.

By taking on these preventive measures and integrating them into your way of life, you can decrease the gamble of dementia and advance cerebrum wellbeing and mental capability over the course of life. Prioritize these strategies to ensure a healthier and more fulfilling future because it is never too late to start making positive changes for your brain health. progressing research and arising intercessions for dementia counteraction.

The field of dementia prevention research is always changing, with new approaches and promising developments.
The following are some potential interventions and key areas of focus:

1. Interventions in one's lifestyle: - Research keeps on investigating the effect of way of life factors like eating regimen, work out, mental feeling, and social commitment on dementia risk. Studies recommend that embracing a mix of solid way of life propensities might assist with decreasing the gamble of mental degradation and dementia.

- Intercessions, for example, multidomain way of life mediations, which consolidate various way of life factors (e.g., diet, work out, mental preparation) at the same time, are being examined for their capability to forestall or defer mental impedance.

2. Healthful Interventions:

- Studies are researching the job of explicit supplements and dietary examples in advancing cerebrum wellbeing and lessening the gamble of dementia. The Mediterranean diet, for instance, has been linked to a lower risk of dementia and cognitive decline due to its emphasis on whole grains, fish, and healthy fats.

- Research is progressing to recognize dietary enhancements and healthful intercessions that might uphold mental capability and lessen the gamble of dementia, like omega-3 unsaturated fats, cancer prevention agents, and vitamin D.

3. Actual work Interventions:

- Actual work intercessions, including high-impact work out, obstruction preparing, and balance works out, are being read up for their capability to work on mental capability and diminish the gamble of dementia. Exercise may have neuroprotective effects on the brain, promoting neuroplasticity, neurogenesis, and the release of neurotrophic factors that support cognitive function and brain health, according to recent research.

4. Brain stimulation and cognitive training: - It is being looked into whether cognitive training interventions, such as memory training, reasoning exercises, and computer-based cognitive programs, can improve cognitive function and lower the risk of dementia.

- Painless mind excitement methods, for example, transcranial attractive feeling (TMS) and transcranial direct current excitement (tDCS) are being explored for their capability to adjust cerebrum movement and work on mental capability in people in danger of dementia.

5. Pharmacological Interventions:

Drugs that target underlying disease mechanisms like neuroinflammation, oxidative stress, and the accumulation of amyloid-beta and tau proteins are the focus of ongoing research into pharmacological interventions for the prevention of dementia. Monoclonal antibodies, small molecule inhibitors, and immunotherapies are some of the potential treatments being tested in clinical trials to slow or stop the progression of Alzheimer's disease and other forms of dementia.

6.Multi-modal and combination therapies: - Scientists are investigating the possible advantages of mix treatments and multimodal approaches that focus on numerous pathways engaged with dementia pathogenesis. These strategies aim to maximize therapeutic effects and improve

outcomes for individuals at risk of dementia by combining lifestyle interventions, pharmacological treatments, and other approaches.

In general, scientists, clinicians, public health specialists, and policymakers collaborate on ongoing research into dementia prevention. Researchers hope to lessen the global burden of dementia and enhance brain health and cognitive function for people all over the world by expanding our knowledge of the intricate mechanisms that underlie dementia and identifying effective preventive measures. Making proactive strides towards cerebrum wellbeing is one of the most enabling things you can accomplish for yourself.

To encourage you to make brain health a priority,

1. Strengthening through Knowledge: By finding out about the elements that impact cerebrum wellbeing and mental capability, you gain the ability to pursue informed decisions that can emphatically influence your mind wellbeing and by and large prosperity.

2. Interest in Your Future: Very much like keeping up with actual wellbeing, putting resources into mind wellbeing is an interest in your future self. By making proactive strides now, you might possibly diminish the gamble of mental degradation and partake in a greater of life as you age.

3. Celebration of Progress: Celebrate the progress you make along the way, whether it's changing your habits to be healthier, finishing cognitive exercises, or reaching personal goals. It's a victory that deserves to be congratulated for each step you take toward better brain health.

4. Keep in Mind the Long-Term Benefits:

Keep in mind that putting brain health first has long-term benefits. By sustaining your cerebrum through solid way of life decisions, you're establishing the groundwork for long haul mental strength and prosperity.

5. Association with Your Objectives and Values: Think about how focusing on mind wellbeing lines up with your own objectives and values. Whether it's keeping up with freedom, remaining intellectually sharp, or getting a charge out of significant connections, dealing with your cerebrum can assist you with carrying on with a day to day existence lined up with what makes the biggest difference to you.

6. Motivation from Others: Draw motivation from people who have focused on cerebrum wellbeing and seen positive results. Seeing the results of proactive brain health practices and hearing success stories can inspire you to take action in your own life.

7. Potential for Development and Adaptation: Recall that the mind is surprisingly versatile and fit for change over the course of life. By taking part in exercises that test and animate your mind, you can advance brain adaptability and upgrade mental capability at whatever stage in life.

8. Little Advances Lead to Enormous Results:

Even little changes in way of life propensities can essentially affect mind wellbeing after some time. Center around approaching slowly and carefully and gathering speed progressively towards a better mind and a more promising time to come.

9. Taking care of oneself and Well-Being:

Focusing on mind wellbeing is a demonstration of taking care of oneself and self-empathy. By sustaining your mind, you're supporting your general prosperity and upgrading your capacity to carry on with a satisfying and significant life.

10. You Merit the Best: At last, recall that you have the right to appreciate ideal cerebrum wellbeing and mental capability. By focusing on yourself and making proactive strides towards mind wellbeing, you're putting resources into your own bliss, satisfaction, and life span.

In this way, embrace the excursion towards better cerebrum wellbeing with energy, assurance, and a feeling of probability. Your mind is a valuable asset, and via really focusing on it, you're preparing for a more brilliant, more energetic future.

Conclusion

Significance of Dementia Prevention Dementia counteraction is critical for protecting mental capability, keeping up with freedom, and working on generally speaking personal satisfaction. By taking on proactive methodologies to help cerebrum wellbeing, people can lessen their gamble of mental degradation and postpone the beginning of dementia.

Methodologies for Dementia Prevention:

1. Sound Way of life Habits:

- Follow a fair eating routine wealthy in natural products, vegetables, entire grains, lean proteins, and solid fats.
- Be physically active on a regular basis, aiming for 150 minutes of moderate exercise per week.
- Avoid smoking, keep your alcohol intake to a minimum, and effectively manage stress.

2. Mental Stimulation:

- Remain intellectually dynamic by participating in mentally animating exercises like perusing, riddles, games, and mastering new abilities. - Engage in brain-challenging hobbies and pursuits as well as opportunities for lifelong learning.

3. Social Engagement:

- Through regular interactions, outings, and group activities, you can keep your social connections with friends, family, and peers.
- Volunteer, join clubs or local area associations, and partake in get-togethers to

cultivate significant connections and battle social disconnection.

4. Quality of Sleep:

 - Focus on quality rest by laying out a standard rest plan, pursuing great rest cleanliness routines, and making a loosening up sleep time schedule.
 - Guarantee satisfactory rest and revival for ideal mind capability and by and large prosperity.

5. Stress Reduction:

 - Practice pressure decrease methods like care, reflection, profound breathing activities, and unwinding procedures to advance close to home prosperity and lessen the gamble of ongoing pressure.

6. Standard Medical services Monitoring:

 - Go to customary check-ups with medical services suppliers to screen generally wellbeing, evaluate mental capability, and talk about any worries or changes in memory or thinking. For the purpose of early detection and treatment of conditions that may raise the risk of dementia, adhere to medical advice and screening recommendations. By carrying out these systems into day to day existence, people can make proactive strides towards keeping up with cerebrum wellbeing, decreasing the gamble of mental deterioration, and advancing in general prosperity. Dementia counteraction is a long lasting excursion that requires responsibility, however the advantages of protecting mental capability and partaking in a more excellent of life put forth it definitely worth the attempt.

Dear reader ,

Leaving on the excursion towards better cerebrum wellbeing is a brave and engaging choice. By making proactive way of life changes and looking for help from medical care experts, you are assuming responsibility for your prosperity and putting resources into a more promising time to come for yourself.

Executing Way of life Changes: It's memorable's essential that each little step you take towards a better way of life is a triumph worth celebrating. Whether it's integrating more leafy foods into your eating regimen, beginning another work-out daily schedule, or rehearsing care and stress-decrease strategies, every decision you make adds to your general mind wellbeing and essentialness.

Believe in your own adaptability: Have faith in your capacity to roll out sure improvements and confidence simultaneously. Recollect that progress may not generally be direct, and mishaps are a characteristic piece of the excursion. What makes the biggest difference is your obligation to your wellbeing and your eagerness to continue to push ahead, slowly and carefully. Looking for Help from Medical services Professionals:

Your medical services group is here to help you constantly. Go ahead and out for direction, counsel, and support. Whether it's booking normal check-ups, examining worries about mental capability, or investigating treatment choices, your medical services supplier is an important partner as you continued looking for better mind wellbeing.

You Are Not Alone: Recollect that you are in good company on this excursion. Companions, family, and friends can offer important help, consolation, and responsibility as you pursue your objectives. Share your goals, praise your victories, and rest on others for help when required.

Your Wellbeing Matters: Your wellbeing and prosperity are valuable gifts, meriting care, consideration, and sustaining. By focusing on your mind wellbeing, you are putting resources into a future loaded up with imperativeness, lucidity, and happiness. Your endeavors today will establish the groundwork for a long period of mental flexibility and prosperity.

Take the Main Step: The excursion towards better mind wellbeing starts with a solitary step. Make that stride today, realizing that you have the strength, assurance, and backing you want to succeed. Have faith in yourself, trust all the while, and embrace the extraordinary force of positive change.

You Can Do This: You deserve a life of health, happiness, and fulfillment because you are capable, resilient, and deserving. Trust in your capacity to make the existence you imagine, and realize that you have all that you want to prevail inside you. You are more grounded than you know, and you can do this.

Sincerely, determination, and backing, you can accomplish your objectives and make the dynamic, satisfying life you merit. Venture out today, and let your excursion towards better mind wellbeing start. **You got this!**